DIABETES

Diabetes Prevention And Symptoms Reversing

Guide To Diabetes Diet, Nutrition Tips, The "Cure" For Diabetes Type 2

BY SANDRA WILLIAMS

Table of Contents

Introduction 4

    [Your Free Gift] 5

Chapter 1: Important Statistics on Diabetes 8

Chapter 2: What Are The Common Symptoms Of Diabetes 10

Chapter 3: Checking Blood Sugar Levels 15

    What do your results mean? 17

Chapter 4: Can You Reverse Type II Diabetes? 18

Chapter 5: What Has Nutrition Got To Do With It? 20

    How to include sweets in your diet? 23

    How to cut down on sugar? 24

Chapter 6: What About Exercise? 28

Conclusion 31

    Would you like to know more? 32

[BONUS] 33

    Preview of my other book, Wheat Belly Diet 33

    Check out my other books 35

Introduction

I want to thank you and congratulate you for purchasing the book *"Diabetes - Diabetes Prevention And Symptoms Reversing"*. This book contains all the information you need to know about managing Diabetes from what to eat, what to avoid, and how to address diabetes symptoms.

For many people, being diagnosed with diabetes is like a death sentence. The simple fact that you know that the condition can kill you, if you don't take caution, is enough to give you sleepless nights. However, this does not need to be so. Just because you are diabetic does not mean that you cannot live and enjoy life. All that you need to do is be more careful in terms of what you eat, when you eat, as well as how and when you exercise. This is not hard at all considering that all of us, whether diabetic or not, need to pay attention to what we eat and our exercise regime, if we don't want to end up overweight or obese.

This book has lots of valuable information about diabetics. You will learn how to reverse diabetic symptoms and what you should eat in order to live a healthy complication-free life. You will also find a very helpful and easy to follow guide to diabetes diet. Reading this book will give you a sort of new lease of life because you will learn that living with diabetes does not need to be as hard as many people take it to be.

Thanks again for getting this book, I hope you will enjoy it!

PS. Looking for a meal plan? Check out the book ***Diabetic Cookbook***, it's full of delicious recipes specifically prepared for diabetics. Get it from Amazon here: http://bit.ly/diabetic-cookbook

[Your Free Gift]

As a way of saying thanks for your purchase, I'm offering 2 gifts that are exclusive to my readers:

To watch a video on How To Defeat Diabetes Forever, go here:

=> http://projecteasylife.com/defeating-diabetes-kit <=

To check what are The 101 Tips That Burn Belly Fat Daily, go to my page here:

=> http://projecteasylife.com/101tips <=

© **Copyright 2015 by Sandra Williams - All rights reserved.**

This document is geared towards providing exact and reliable information in regards to the topic and issue covered. The publication is sold with the idea that the publisher is not required to render accounting, officially permitted, or otherwise, qualified services. If advice is necessary, legal or professional, a practiced individual in the profession should be ordered.

From a Declaration of Principles which was accepted and approved equally by a Committee of the American Bar Association and a Committee of Publishers and Associations.

In no way is it legal to reproduce, duplicate, or transmit any part of this document in either electronic means or in printed format. Recording of this publication is strictly prohibited and any storage of this document is not allowed unless with written permission from the publisher. All rights reserved.

The information provided herein is stated to be truthful and consistent, in that any liability, in terms of inattention or otherwise, by any usage or abuse of any policies, processes, or directions contained within is the solitary and utter responsibility of the recipient reader. Under no circumstances will any legal responsibility or blame be held against the publisher for any reparation, damages, or monetary loss due to the information herein, either directly or indirectly.

Respective authors own all copyrights not held by the publisher.

The information herein is offered for informational purposes solely, and is universal as so. The presentation of the information is without contract or any type of guarantee assurance.

The trademarks that are used are without any consent, and the publication of the trademark is without permission or backing by the trademark owner. All trademarks and brands within this book are for clarifying purposes only and are the owned by the owners themselves, not affiliated with this document.

DISCLAIMER: The purpose of this book is to provide information only. The information, though believed to be entirely accurate, is NOT a substitution for medical, psychological or professional advice, diagnosis or treatment. The author recommends that you seek the advice of your physician or other qualified health care provider to present them with questions you may have regarding any medical condition. Advice from your trusted, professional medical advisor should always supersede information presented in this book.

Chapter 1: Important Statistics on Diabetes

The importance of living a healthy lifestyle cannot be overemphasized, and yet the number of blood sugar and heart related diseases continues to increase on a daily basis. More than 29 million U.S citizens have diabetes today, up from the estimated 26 million back in 2010. Of these, 1 in every 4 people do not know they have it. 86 million more adults in the United States have pre-diabetes, a state in which your blood sugar levels are higher than usual, but not high enough to be considered type 2 diabetes. Without moderate physical activity and weight regulation, 15 to 30 percent of these people will eventually develop type 2 diabetes in five years' time.

About 2 years ago, Anne Tierney was devastated to learn that she had type 2 diabetes. Her diagnosis came as a shock, even though she was about forty pounds overweight by then. She used to eat chocolate all the time, but quit immediately after her diagnosis results came out. She also hired a personal trainer and consulted a nutritionist.

If you are diagnosed with diabetes, like in Anne Tierney's case, taking quick action is always the best. The main reason why a huge percentage of people living with type 2 diabetes are unaware they have the disease, is that it is normally diagnosed years after its onset, in which case it would have already done enough damage. The result is serious complications, including kidney disease, heart disease, infections, erectile dysfunction, blindness, and much more. Maintaining normal blood glucose levels may slow or prevent the progress of these complications.

Studies show that more than 80 percent of type 2 diabetes patients are obese, but people find it daunting to even think about losing 40 or 50 pounds. However, losing as little as 10 pounds is sufficient enough to cause a significant impact on your blood sugar levels. There are basically two dietary secrets to achieving this goal: making wise food choices and limiting your portion sizes. Spend some time measuring and weighing your food to know how much you are eating, and try to always read the labels.

Let us look at some common symptoms of diabetes…

Chapter 2: What Are The Common Symptoms Of Diabetes

Type 2 diabetes, once referred to as non-insulin dependent diabetes or adult onset diabetes, is a chronic condition that affects your body's ability to metabolize sugar (glucose), which is the most important source of fuel for your body. The condition causes your body to resist the effects of insulin, the hormone that enhances movement of sugar into your cells. It can also hinder the production of sufficient insulin in your body, leading to an imbalance in glucose levels. While type II diabetes is more prevalent in adults, it is now affecting children especially with the increasing child obesity cases. There is also no known cure, but you can control the symptoms by eating well, maintaining a healthy weight, and exercising. If you are not 100 percent sure if you have diabetes, you may want to check out for these symptoms:

Increased urination and constant thirst

If you frequently need to urinate, you may be suffering from diabetes. Your kidneys are very active and strive to eliminate all the extra glucose in your blood, thus the frequent urge to relieve yourself. The excessive thirst is an indication that your body is trying to regain the lost fluids. These two symptoms appear simultaneously, and are some of the ways your body tries to manage high blood sugar.

Weight loss

Ridiculously high levels of blood sugar can also lead to rapid weight loss. This could be approximately 10-20 pounds over a period of 2 to 3 months, but not in a healthy way. Since the insulin hormone is not doing its work of moving glucose into your cells to be used as energy, your body thinks it is starving, and triggers the breakdown of protein from your muscles as a secondary source of fuel. Moreover, the kidneys are also in full gear in a bid to get rid of excess sugar, leading to a loss of calories. Since both of these processes require a lot of energy, you end up creating a calorie deficit.

Hunger

Extreme hunger pangs are another symptom of diabetes that occurs as a result of sharp peaks of highs and lows in your blood sugar levels. Your body naturally assumes it has not been fed once your blood sugar levels plummet, which makes it crave for the glucose necessary for the cells to function.

Skin problems

You may also experience itchy skin, perhaps due to poor circulation or dry skin. Acanthosis Nigricans is also a skin condition associated with type 2 diabetes. It is a condition characterized by the darkening of skin, around the armpit or neck area. If you have this condition, you probably also have insulin resistance, even though your blood sugar might not be high.

Yeast infections

Experts consider diabetes an immune-suppressed state, which simply means heightened vulnerability to a variety of infections, the most common of them being yeast and other fungal infections. Both fungi and bacteria thrive in sugar rich surroundings. Women, in particular, should keep an eye for vaginal candida infections.

Slow healing

Cuts, bruises and infections that are persistent are a classic sign of diabetes. This is normally due to the excess glucose moving through the veins and arteries, ultimately damaging your blood vessels. This makes it difficult for blood to reach different parts of your body to facilitate healing.

Blurry vision

Seeing occasional flashes of light, or floaters and having distorted vision are often directly linked to high levels of blood sugar. Blurry vision is caused by a refraction problem. High blood sugar levels tend to change the shape of the eye and lens. Fortunately, you can reverse this symptom once you get your blood sugar levels back to normal or near normal. On the other hand, neglecting to check your blood sugar levels for a long time will lead the glucose to causing permanent damage, perhaps even blindness, and that is not reversible.

Fatigue and irritability

People who have had high blood sugar levels for a long time tend to get used to persistently not feeling well. This often makes them to be constantly visiting their doctor. Getting up several times to go to the bathroom during the night is enough to make anyone tired, as well as the additional effort your body expends to compensate for its glucose deficiency. Irritability breeds from tiredness. It is not uncommon for people whose blood sugar levels have been really high to acknowledge that they didn't realize how bad they felt as soon as their blood sugar levels are brought down.

Tingling or numbness

If you experience tingling or numbness in your hands and feet, followed by swelling or burning pain, this is a sign that your nerves are being attacked by diabetes. If the symptoms are recent, you may be able to reverse it. However, just like with vision, if you allow your blood sugar levels to be high for too long, neuropathy will be permanent.

Blood tests

You can also check for diabetes using several tests, but a single test result is not enough to diagnose the condition. The fasting plasma glucose test is one such test, which involves checking your blood sugar levels after 8 hours or a night of not eating. If two of these tests show that your blood glucose is above 126 mg/dL, it means you have diabetes. 99 mg/dL is the normal cutoff, while 100 to 125 mg/dL blood glucose is considered pre-diabetes.

What happens when you suspect that you are diabetic after noticing that you have some of the symptoms mentioned above? Well, the best way to go about that is to check your blood sugar levels to ensure that they are in check.

Chapter 3: Checking Blood Sugar Levels

When your body is functioning normally, it automatically checks your blood glucose levels. If it is too high or too low, it adjusts the levels to return to normal. On the other hand, when you have diabetes, your body lacks the ability to regulate your blood glucose automatically, which essentially means you have to check your blood sugar regularly and adjust your treatment accordingly. A doctor can measure your blood sugar levels during an office visit. Nevertheless, the truth is that the levels change on an hourly basis, which means visiting the doctor only every few weeks will not show you your daily blood glucose levels. DIY tests help people with diabetes measure their blood glucose daily. A urine test is the easiest test you can do at home. When your blood glucose levels rise above normal, the excess is gotten rid of by the kidneys in form of urine, thereby reflecting an excess of glucose in your blood.

Taking a urine test is easy. You just dip the tablets or paper strips in urine, and then check for the color change that will determine whether your blood glucose is too high. The urine test is however, not entirely accurate since it only reflects the level of blood glucose some hours earlier. Moreover, everyone's kidneys are not the same. The concentration of glucose in two given people may be the same, but their sugar levels can be different. Its accuracy can further be complicated by certain drugs and vitamin C. The most accurate way to measure blood glucose accurately is to do it directly using kits.

You basically prick a finger to draw a drop of blood using a spring operated lancet. You then place the drop of blood on a strip of specially coated plastic or small machines that tell you how much blood glucose is in your blood. It is generally advisable to test your blood glucose levels several times a day. Monitoring your blood glucose can show you how your body responds to diabetes treatment, stress, exercise and meals.

A glycosylated hemoglobin test is another test used to measure the effectiveness of treatment. It measures the amount of glucose that has been attached to hemoglobin, the pigment in your red blood cells that gives your blood its red color. Hemoglobin absorbs glucose over time, depending on its concentration in your blood. Once it has been absorbed by hemoglobin, the glucose stays there until the blood cells die and are replaced by new ones. A doctor can determine whether your blood glucose has been very high over the last couple of months, using the glycosylated hemoglobin test.

What are the target ranges?

The blood glucose targets are specified, depending on:

- Duration of diabetes
- Comorbid conditions
- Age and life expectancy
- Individual patient considerations
- Hypoglycemia unawareness
- Advanced microvascular complications or known CVD

The following targets are recommended for most non-pregnant adults with type 2 diabetes.

- AIC – 7 percent
- Pre-prandial plasma glucose before a meal – 70 to 130 mg/dL
- Post-prandial plasma glucose – 1 to 2 hours after starting the meal – Less than 180 mg/dL

What do your results mean?

Write down your blood glucose test results once you are done, and then review them to see how stress, food, and activity affect your blood glucose. Monitor your blood sugar levels for several days in a row at about the same time, and then check the record to see if the levels are too high or too low. Keep in mind that these numbers can trigger strong feelings. Your blood glucose results can leave you feeling down, angry, frustrated, confused or upset. It is easy to judge yourself from the numbers. Remember that your blood glucose levels are a way to monitor how well your care plan is working. The results may be an indication that you need to change your diabetes plan.

After understanding the results, the next thing is to formulate a plan on how to live with diabetes. This plan should have in mind whether you can actually reverse diabetes. Let us see this in the following chapter.

Chapter 4: Can You Reverse Type II Diabetes?

It sounds too good to be true, doesn't it? Can you actually reverse type II diabetes through healthy eating and exercise? Certain lifestyle changes have been proven crucial in managing diabetes, but whether you can actually turn back the hands of time to a state where you never had diabetes at all is another matter. It all depends on how long you have had the condition, its severity, and your genes. The word reversal as far as diabetes control is concerned is a term used to describe the steps taken to manage the condition to a point where you no longer need medication, but still have to engage in a healthy lifestyle to stay that way. Health professionals usually refer to type 2 diabetes as a chronic and progressive illness. Now, this may sound like a paradox, considering that chronic means you will always have the disease, and progressive means it will almost certainly get worse. This may leave you wondering, if it only gets worse, if you cannot avoid complications and premature death, then why should you bother with your diet to manage diabetes?

Although the condition has been branded a chronic and progressive disease, several people living with diabetes beg to differ. A study was conducted where eleven subjects were put on a 600 calories diet, and after 8 weeks they had regained normal insulin function, stopped taking their medicines, and had normal lab results. While it has long been believed that type 2 diabetes is irreversible, times have changed, and studies have shown that we can reverse the condition. Moreover, starvation is not the only way to reverse type 2 diabetes. You don't need an extreme diet, or you don't necessarily have to lose weight, and you most definitely don't need surgery. Just drastically reducing or cutting out starches and sugars, and working out more can reverse type II diabetes in about 80 percent of patients.

Let us look at how you can actually manage diabetes and even reverse the condition.

Chapter 5: What Has Nutrition Got To Do With It?

Type 2 diabetes is a lifestyle condition. The food you eat can either promote or prevent insulin resistance and subsequent diabetes. To prevent or reverse type 2 diabetes and enhance healthy insulin sensitivity, actual anti-diabetes foods have to minimize blood glucose highs and maximize phyto-chemical value.

Scientists have long discovered a link between nutrition and the incidence of type 2 diabetes. For instance, when you eat too much added sugar, your pancreas releases high amounts of the hormone insulin to get rid of the excess sugar. Taking too much sugar on a regular basis can offset a cascade of metabolic disturbances like insulin resistance, which inevitably leads to type 2 diabetes. Studies have also shown that excessive sugar intake can increase your risk of diabetes, regardless of other factors such as alcohol consumption, calorie intake and obesity. Let us look at what you can eat in order to deal with diabetes and even reverse its symptoms.

Go for high fiber, slow release carbs

You may not know this, but carbohydrates greatly affect your blood sugar levels, more than fats and proteins. The good news is that you don't have to avoid them completely. You only have to be selective about the types of carbohydrates you take. It is generally best to limit highly refined carbohydrates such as white bread, rice and pasta, as well as soda, snack foods and candy. Rather, focus on high fiber complex carbohydrates, otherwise known as slow release carbohydrates. These carbohydrates help maintain blood sugar levels at normal standards because they take longer to be digested, thus preventing the production of excess insulin in your body. They are also a great source of long lasting energy, and will keep you feeling full for longer. Substitute the following foods on the left with the ones on the right:

- White rice – brown or wild rice

- Regular pasta – whole wheat pasta

- White potatoes – sweet potatoes, cauliflower mash, winter squash, yams

- White bread – whole grain or whole wheat bread

- Instant oatmeal – rolled or steel cut oats

- Sugary breakfast cereal – high fiber breakfast cereal such as raising bran

- Cornflakes – bran flakes

The glycemic index shows you the speed at which your system turns food into sugar. Glycemic load, on the other hand, shows both your glycemic index and carbohydrate content in a food, thus giving you a clear picture of how a certain food can affect your blood sugar level. High glycemic foods spike your blood sugar levels rapidly, while low ones have the least effect. You don't have to go online to check glycemic index and glycemic load tables; there is an easier way to regulate the carbohydrates you eat. Foods can be classified into three broad categories: coal, water and fire. The more work your body has to do in order to break down food, the better.

- Fire foods: These have a high glycemic index, and are low in protein and fiber. Examples include foods such as white bread, potatoes, white pasta, white rice, and most baked foods, chips, sweets and most processed foods. You should limit these in your diet.

- Water foods: These are free foods, meaning that you can eat as much of them as you wish. They include all vegetables and most fruits. However, dried fruit, canned fruit packed in syrup, and fruit juice spike blood sugar rapidly and do not fall under this category.
- Coal foods: These have a low glycemic index, and are rich in protein and fiber. Examples include lean meats, nuts & seeds, beans and whole grains like whole wheat pasta, whole wheat bread and brown rice.

Studies have shown that the key to weight regulation is to reduce the amount of refined carbohydrates in your diet. Focus instead on the "coal" or low GI foods, which will keep you feeling fuller for longer. These foods are digested slowly in your body, thus slowing the absorption of sugar into your bloodstream. The result is that you are less likely to experience a rise in your blood sugar levels, you will feel satiated for longer, and will not likely overeat. Steer away from processed foods such as sugary desserts, baked goods, and packaged cereal, and instead go for beans, steel cut oats, whole grains, dark green leafy vegetables, and fat free yogurt. In addition, eat whole fresh fruit, rather than fruit juice.

Be smart about sweets and sugar

Eating for diabetes does not necessarily mean eliminating sugar. You can still enjoy your favorite dessert occasionally if you have diabetes. While most sugar addicts generally have a sweet tooth, and find cutting back on sweets almost as bad as eliminating them altogether, you may be comforted to know that cravings do disappear, and preferences change. As you incorporate healthy eating habits, you may find that the foods you used to enjoy now seem too sweet or too rich.

How to include sweets in your diet?

- Hold back on the bread, pasta or rice if you want dessert. Including sweets in a meal adds more carbohydrates, thus the reason to cut back on the other carbohydrate foods in the meal.

- Include some healthy fat in your dessert. It may sound counterintuitive to go for high fat desserts over the low fat or fat free ones, but fat slows down digestion, which means your blood sugar levels will not spike as rapidly. However, you should insist on eating healthy fats like olive oil, coconut oil and flaxseed oil, especially the cold pressed ones.

- Savor each bite when eating dessert. If you are like most people, you have probably mindlessly eaten your way through a huge piece of cake or a bag of cookies countless times. Can you actually say that you enjoyed every bite? Indulge yourself in the food by eating slowly and paying close attention to its textures and flavors. This will prevent you from overeating, and you will enjoy it much more.

How to cut down on sugar?

- Reduce the amount of juice, soda and soft drinks you take. A recent study showed that for every 12 ounce serving of a sweetened beverage you take every day, you increase your risk for diabetes by approximately 15 percent. To get your carbonation kick, try instead sparking water with a splash of fruit juice or a twist of lemon or lime.

- Sweeten your own foods. Go for unsweetened iced tea, unflavored oatmeal or plain yogurt and then add a sweetener for yourself. Most manufacturers tend to go overboard when adding sweeteners.

- Cut back on the amount of sugar in your recipes by a quarter or a third. For example, instead of using 1 cup of sugar in a given recipe, go for 2/3 or ¾ cup.

- Find healthier ways to satisfy your cravings. Rather than going for ice cream, blend frozen bananas instead for a creamy, frozen treat. On the other hand, instead of taking your usual milk chocolate bar, enjoy a small piece of dark chocolate.

- Eat half of your normal dessert, and then replace the other half with a fruit.

It is also easy to underestimate the amount of carbohydrates and calories in alcoholic drinks, including wine and beer. Cocktails mixed with juice and sugar in particular, tend to be loaded with sugar. If you must drink, then do so in moderation. That is to say, no more than 2 (12-ounce) drinks for men, and 1 (12-ounce) for women. In addition, go for calorie free drinks, and only drink when eating. If you already have diabetes, it is crucial that you monitor your blood glucose because alcohol can interfere with insulin sensitivity and diabetes medication.

Choose fats wisely

Depending on the type, fats can either be harmful or helpful in your diet. You are at a higher risk of heart disease if you are diabetic, hence the need to be smart about your fats. There are basically two types of fats: healthy and unhealthy fats. However, all fats are high in calories, so it is advisable to watch your portion sizes as well. Saturated fats and trans fats are the two most destructive fats. The main source of saturated fats is animal products such as whole milk dairy products and red meat. On the other hand, trans fats, also referred to as partially hydrogenated oils, are formed when hydrogen is added to liquid vegetables to solidify them and prolong their lifespan. While this is marvelous news for manufacturers, the opposite can be said for you. Unsaturated fats are the best fats. The main sources are fish and plants. Unsaturated fats are liquid at room temperature. The best examples include avocados, nuts, canola oil, and olive oil. Eat more of omega 3 fatty acids as well, as these are highly effective in supporting brain & heart health, as well as in fighting inflammation. Excellent sources include flaxseeds, tuna and salmon.

You can reduce unhealthy fats in your diet and add healthy fats by:

- Substituting your regular vegetable oil or butter with olive oil.

- Trimming any visible fat from meat before cooking and removing the skin from your turkey and chicken before cooking.

- Snacking on seeds or nuts instead of chips and crackers. For a filling snack, have a healthy handful or include them in your morning cereal. Nut butters are also full of healthy fats and are very satisfying.

- Grilling, boiling, baking and stir frying instead of frying.

- Serving fish 2 to 3 times per week instead of red meat.

- Adding avocado to your sandwiches, as opposed to cheese; the creamy texture will still be there, but the health factor will improve.

- Using applesauce or canola oil when baking, as opposed to shortening or butter.

- Preparing your soups with low fat milk thickened with pureed potatoes, flour, or reduced fat sour cream instead of using heavy cream.

Eat regularly and keep a food diary

If you are overweight, the good news is that you only have to shed about 7 percent of your overall body weight in order to reduce your risk of diabetes by half. Moreover, you don't even have to count your calories obsessively or starve yourself to achieve this. As far as successful weight loss is concerned, research has shown that two of the most effective strategies involve recording what you eat, and adhering to a regular eating schedule. Your body has an easier time regulating your blood sugar levels and weight when you follow a regular meal schedule. Plan to eat moderate and consistent portions for every meal and snack.

In addition:

- Avoid skipping breakfast, start off your day with a healthy and heavy breakfast. This will provide you with enough energy for the day, as well as help you maintain steady blood sugar levels.

- Eat small, regular meals – maximum of 6 every day: People tend to overeat when they are excessively hungry, so eating small, regular meals can help you monitor your portions.

- Maintain constant calorie intake: Monitoring the amount of calories you eat on a daily basis can have an impact on the consistency of your blood sugar levels. Try eating approximately the same amount of calories every day.

Research has also shown that people who keep a food journal when trying to lose weight have a higher probability of achieving their goal, and keeping it that way. In fact, keeping a food diary can actually help you lose twice as much weight as you would have without doing so. But how does putting down what you eat and drink on paper help you shed more pounds? For starters, it shows you your problem areas, such as your morning latte or your afternoon snack i.e. where you are getting excess calories than expected. It also makes you aware of what, why and how much you are eating, which ultimately helps you cut back on emotional eating and mindless snacking.

Chapter 6: What About Exercise?

You may consider exercise a chore, a nuisance, or simply a bore, but if you have been diagnosed with type II diabetes, you have no choice but to look at it in a whole new light. Physical activity is a tool in itself. Just like altering your diet or taking medication, exercise can lower your blood glucose on its own, even without losing weight. In fact, exercise is one of the most underused treatments, and it is very powerful. If you are a diabetic or are looking to prevent its onset, exercising is a safe and highly recommended way to reduce your risk of other complications. However, you may want to check with your doctor to ascertain you do not have heart problems, nerve damage, or any other issue that needs special consideration when working out.

Generally, your blood sugar levels drop after exercising, and remain lower for the next 24 – 48 hours. Exercise makes your muscles more sensitive to insulin, thereby absorbing more glucose from the blood. However, like many type 2 diabetes aspects, the response can be highly individualized. Sometimes, exercise can boost blood sugar. When starting, you will need to test your blood glucose levels before, during, and after exercise to check how your body is responding. Exercise also plays a major role in lowering blood pressure, which is very beneficial, considering that high blood pressure can lead to heart attacks, eye problems, strokes, kidney failure, and other complications associated with type 2 diabetes.

Most experts agree that you should exercise at least five days a week. Each session should last not less than 30 minutes, and should be of moderate intensity. Here are excellent examples of moderate intensity exercise you can do:

- Fast walking
- Cycling at 5 to 9mph
- Swimming
- Rowing
- Dancing
- Mowing the lawn

When doing these kinds of exercises, you should experience an increase in your breathing rate, as well as your heart rate. You should also burn about 3.5 – 7 calories per minute, and reach a METs of 3-6 (MET is the acronym for Metabolic Equivalent). You have a MET of 1 when you are sitting down and doing nothing. Walking slowly can make your MET rise to 2 or 2.5. Walking normally can raise your MET to 3, while a brisk walk on the other hand can bring it to 5. If an stray lion suddenly appeared in the street in front of you and started chasing you, your desperate sprint would boost your MET up to 8 or 9!

If it has been long since you exercised, you may want to take it slow and start with light exercise, and then build up slowly with time. Add a little time to every session after each week, and/or increase the intensity. Keep in mind that regular exercise is all that matters. For example, 5 days of 30 minutes' exercise is way better than 1 day of 150 minutes' exercise per week.

Strength training has also been shown to be great in regulating diabetes, especially because strength training exercises help you build muscles.

Several gyms today have qualified and experienced trainers/staff to deal with people with various conditions and illnesses. Having someone accompany you, and push you along occasionally can be a great motivator. Gyms are all rounded. You will find equipment to provide you with immediate feedback on how well you are fairing – your heart rate, speed, your progress, calories burnt per minute or hour, and so forth.

The effect of exercise on your blood sugar levels will vary depending on how long you are active and several other factors. As said earlier, exercise can lower your blood sugar and keep it low for the next 24 hours or more by increasing your body's sensitivity to insulin. You should familiarize yourself with how your blood glucose changes during exercise. Checking your blood sugar level several times before and after any physical activity can give you a clue of the benefits of the activity. You can also keep a record of your body's reaction to various physical activities, and determine how they alter your blood glucose. Being aware of these patterns can help you avoid the highs and lows of your blood glucose.

Exercise can sometimes cause a rise in blood sugar levels, and this is known as hyperglycemia. Avoid any form of exercise if your blood glucose concentration is above 300 mg/dL, and your urine has traces of ketones. Always check your blood glucose level before and after exercise to see how it has been affected by exercise. If you have diabetic retinopathy, a condition characterized by damaged blood vessels in the retina of the eye, you may damage your eyesight with exercise. Strenuous activities such as weight lifting and jogging could also cause retinal detachment or bleeding, so you may want to avoid these activities.

Conclusion

Thank you again for purchasing this book!

As earlier indicated, being diagnosed with diabetes is not a death sentence. With proper diet and exercise and suitable lifestyle, you are well on your way to reversing diabetes. Always remember that you have to start somewhere so even though it may seem difficult at the beginning, remember that it will get better with time and as you continue in consistency, you will feel better with each passing day until you feel new again and as though you never had diabetes!

I hope this book has been of great help in providing the information you needed regarding being able to successfully manage diabetes symptoms as well as reverse the condition. Remember that it is never too late to start so start doing something now and enjoy the benefits.

Now I would like to ask for a *small* favor. I am self-published author, and if you liked my book, a review on Amazon would be a great help for me. This feedback will let me continue to write the kind of books that will help people and will let me improve.

Go to http://bit.ly/diabetesreview to review, and thanks in advance for any kind of support!

Thank you and good luck!

– *Sandra*

Would you like to know more?

To watch a video on How To Defeat Diabetes Forever, go here:

=> http://projecteasylife.com/defeating-diabetes-kit <=

To check what are The 101 Tips That Burn Belly Fat Daily, go to my page here:

=> http://projecteasylife.com/101tips <=

[BONUS]

Preview of my other book, Wheat Belly Diet

(…)

Why Use the Wheat Belly Diet for the Best Results?

If you have tried and failed with other diets, perhaps you were not eliminating the right types of foods. Rethinking wheat has helped people to eliminate the harm it causes to your body. Getting rid of belly fat has thus far been a successful goal for people using the Wheat-Belly Diet.

Very few wheat-based foods are actually healthy for you to eat. The wheat used today, which Dr. Davis calls "Frankenwheat", is genetically modified, and it isn't the same wheat that your parents used to eat.

The modification of the wheat plant has allowed it to be thicker and shorter, so that it is more beneficial for farmers, and more resistant to disease. The bad aspect of this wheat is that it is not as nutritionally rich as conventional wheat, and can damage your health.

The glycemic index is higher in today's wheat than it is in sugar. Some candy bars have a healthier glycemic index than a slice of wheat bread. Glutens that are present in larger amounts in today's wheat cause cravings, and that leads to excess belly fat.

Dr. Davis says that you can expect better results from a wheat-free meal plan, because wheat is more than simply a gluten source. "Frankenwheat" affects the mind, by stimulating your appetite and it can cause depression and anxiety, especially for people who are overweight.

Giving up wheat will allow you to lose belly fat, and can also help in other health issues, such as those mentioned above. People are finally beginning to see the negative effects of today's wheat on their health, and those who stay with the Wheat Belly Diet often find benefits that they did not even expect.

(…)

To check out the rest of the book *Wheat Belly Diet*, go to Amazon here: http://bit.ly/wheatbellydiet

Check out my other books

Below you'll find some of my other books that are popular on Amazon and Kindle as well. Simply go to the links below to check them out. Alternatively, you can visit my author page on Amazon to see other work done by me:

Author page: http://bit.ly/SandraWilliams

Gluten Free And Wheat Free Total Health Revolution

Wheat Belly Cookbook *– 37 Wheat Free Recipes To Lose The Wheat And Have All-Day Energy* (http://bit.ly/bellycookbook)

Gluten Free *– The Gluten Free Diet For Beginners Guide, What Is Celiac Disease, How To Eat Healthier And Have More Energy* (http://bit.ly/glutenfreebook)

Gluten Free Cookbook *– 30 Healthy And Easy Gluten Free Recipes For Beginners, Gluten Free Diet Plan For A Healthy Lifestyle* (http://bit.ly/gfreecookbook)

How To REALLY Set And Achieve Goals

Goals *– Setting And Achieving S.M.A.R.T. Goals, How To Stay Motivated And Get Everything You Want From Your Life Faster* (http://bit.ly/getsmartgoals)

Prevent And Reverse Diabetes Disease

Diabetic Cookbook *– 30 Diabetes Diet Recipes For Diabetic Living, Control Low Sugar And Reverse Diabetes Naturally* (http://bit.ly/diabetic-cookbook)

Get Healthy, Have More Energy And Live Longer With Natural Paleo And Mediterranean Foods

Paleo – The Paleo Diet For Beginners Guide, Easy And Practical Solution For Weight Loss And Healthy Eating (http://bit.ly/healthypaleo)

Paleo Cookbook – 30 Healthy And Easy Paleo Diet Recipes For Beginners, Start Eating Healthy And Get More Energy With Practical Paleo Approach (http://bit.ly/tastypaleo)

Mediterranean Diet – Easy Guide To Healthy Life With Mediterranean Cuisine, Fast And Natural Weight Loss For Beginners (http://bit.ly/mediterraneanbook)

Mediterranean Diet Cookbook – 30 Healthy And Easy Mediterranean Diet Recipes For Beginners (http://bit.ly/mediterracookbook)

Extremely Fast Weight Loss With Low Carb Approach

Ketogenic Diet – Easy Keto Diet Guide For Healthy Life And Fast Weight Loss, Heal Yourself And Get More Energy With Low Carb Diet (http://bit.ly/ketodietbook)

Ketogenic Diet Cookbook – 30 Keto Diet Recipes For Beginners, Easy Low Carb Plan For A Healthy Lifestyle And Quick Weight Loss (http://bit.ly/ketocookbook)

Atkins Cookbook – 30 Quick And Easy Atkins Diet Recipes For Beginners, Plan Your Low Carb Days With The New Atkins Diet Book (http://bit.ly/atkinscookbook)

Amazing Weight Loss Tips, Tricks And Motivation

Weight Loss – 30 Tips On How To Lose Weight Fast Without Pills Or Surgery, Weight Loss Motivation And Fat Burning Strategies (http://bit.ly/weightlosstipsbook)

Ultimate Guide To Diets – *Choose The Best Diet For Your Body, Live Healthy And Happy Life Without Supplements And Pills* (http://bit.ly/dietsbook)

The Obesity Cure – *How To Lose Weight Fast And Overcome Obesity Forever* (http://bit.ly/obesitybook)

Unique Beauty Tips Every Woman Should Know

Younger Next Month – *Anti-Aging Guide For Women* (http://bit.ly/beyoungerbook)

Hair Care And Hair Growth Solutions – *How To Regrow Your Hair Faster, Hair Loss Treatment And Hair Growth Remedies* (http://bit.ly/haircarebook)

Improve State Of Mind, Defeat Bad Feelings And Be Happy!

Anxiety Workbook – *Free Cure For Anxiety Disorder And Depression Symptoms, Panic Attacks And Social Anxiety Relief Without Medication And Pills* (http://bit.ly/anxietybook)

The Depression Cure – *Depression Self Help Workbook, Cure And Free Yourself From Depression Naturally And For Life* (http://bit.ly/depressioncurebook)

If the links do not work, for whatever reason, you can simply search for the titles on the Amazon website to find them. Best regards!

Printed in Great Britain
by Amazon.co.uk, Ltd.,
Marston Gate.